Brazilian Mounjaro: The Ultimate Weight Loss Elixir

Shed Pounds and Boost Health
Naturally

Hoover Matthews

About the Author

Hoover Matthews is an elite rower, health enthusiast, and wellness researcher with over 30 years of experience in performance optimization, metabolism, and holistic health. As a lifelong athlete, he has studied the science of nutrition, weight loss, and inflammation reduction, using his expertise to help individuals achieve sustainable health transformations.

Passionate about natural remedies and evidence-based wellness strategies, Hoover explores the connection between gut health, metabolism, and superfoods to develop practical solutions for weight management and longevity.

His latest book, *Brazilian Mounjaro: The Ultimate Weight Loss Elixir*, reveals the power of superfoods and natural detox methods to support fat loss, digestion, and overall vitality. His forthcoming book, *The Inflammation Cure: Unlocking the Secrets to Longevity and Wellness*, dives deep into the triggers and causes of inflammation, offering actionable strategies to reduce inflammation, improve health, and extend lifespan.

When he's not writing, Hoover can be found training on the water, running with his dogs, experimenting with superfood recipes, or helping others improve their health and happiness.

Overview

Chapter One

The Origins and Science Behind the Brazilian Mounjaro Drink

The History of Natural Healing Beverages in Brazil

B razil is known for its rich biodiversity, with the Amazon rainforest and vast landscapes providing an abundance of medicinal plants and natural remedies. For centuries, indigenous tribes and local communities have harnessed the power of nature to create drinks and tonics that promote health, longevity, and wellness. Among these traditional remedies, herbal teas, detoxifying infusions, and metabolism-boosting beverages have played a crucial role in maintaining energy levels, digestion, and immune function.

The Brazilian Mounjaro drink is one such beverage that has gained popularity in recent years. It blends powerful, natural ingredients, including **butterfly pea flowers, apple cider vinegar, lemon juice, honey**, **and ginger** into a vibrant and nutrient-rich elixir. While its origins are not tied to one specific indigenous tribe, the drink embodies Brazil's deep-rooted traditions of using nature to heal, cleanse, and nourish the body.

This vibrant drink has gained popularity due to its stunning color transformation and, more importantly, its potential health benefits. But what makes this combination so effective? To understand, we must dive into the science and traditional uses of each ingredient.

Butterfly Pea Flowers: The Antioxidant Powerhouse

Traditionally used in Southeast Asian and Brazilian herbal medicine, butterfly pea flowers are known for their vibrant blue hue and incredible antioxidant properties. These flowers contain anthocyanins, which:

- Help **reduce inflammation** by neutralizing free radicals.

- Support **brain health** and memory retention.

- Promote **skin elasticity** and youthful appearance.

- Aid in **digestive health** by calming the gut lining.

One of the most striking features of butterfly pea tea is its **color-changing effect**—when combined with lemon juice, the deep blue liquid transforms into a beautiful purple, symbolizing the balance between alkalinity and acidity in the body.

Apple Cider Vinegar: The Metabolic Booster

Apple cider vinegar (ACV) has been a staple in natural medicine for centuries. Traditionally used for digestion and detoxification, ACV is known to:

- Help **regulate blood sugar levels**, reducing cravings and preventing insulin spikes.

- Support **gut health** by promoting beneficial bacteria.

- Aid in **fat metabolism**, making it a useful tool for weight management.

- Act as a natural **detoxifier**, helping to flush out toxins from the body.

Scientific studies have shown that consuming ACV before meals can lead to **improved digestion and satiety**, making it a great addition to a weight-loss-friendly routine.

Lemon Juice: The Digestive and Alkalizing Agent

Lemon juice is widely used in traditional medicine for its detoxifying and alkalizing properties. This citrus powerhouse provides:

- A **rich source of vitamin C**, essential for immune support and skin health.

- **Alkalizing effects**, helping to balance the body's pH and reduce acidity.

- **Digestive aid**, stimulating bile production and supporting liver function.

- **Anti-inflammatory benefits**, reducing oxidative stress in the body.

Honey: The Natural Energy Booster

Raw honey has long been considered a natural remedy for numerous ailments. Traditionally used in Brazilian and Ayurvedic medicine, honey is valued for its:

- **Antimicrobial properties**, helping to fight infections and improve immunity.

- **Natural sweetness**, providing an alternative to processed sugars.

- **Energy-boosting effects**, making it an excellent pre-workout drink ingredient.

- **Gut-soothing benefits**, aiding digestion and reducing bloating.

Ginger: The Inflammation Fighter

Ginger has been used in Ayurvedic and traditional Brazilian medicine for thousands of years. This spicy root is packed with bioactive compounds like gingerol, which provide:

- **Powerful anti-inflammatory effects**, reducing joint pain and muscle soreness.

- **Digestive support**, helping with bloating, nausea, and gut health.

- **Metabolism-boosting properties**, increasing calorie burn and fat oxidation.

- **Immune-enhancing benefits**, protecting the body against infections.

Ginger adds a warming and spicy kick to the Brazilian Mounjaro drink, making it even more effective for improving digestion and circulation.

Why This Combination Works

The synergy between these ingredients makes the Brazilian Mounjaro drink a **powerful natural remedy**. The combination of **antioxidants, metabolic boosters, digestive aids, and immune-strengthening compounds** creates a holistic beverage that can:

- Support **weight loss** by improving metabolism and reducing cravings.

- Reduce **inflammation**, which is a root cause of many chronic diseases.

- Aid in **digestion and gut health**, helping maintain a healthy microbiome.

- Promote **overall well-being**, from brain function to skin health.

Why the Brazilian Mounjaro Drink Stands Out

Unlike many **weight loss fads or commercial detox drinks**, the Brazilian Mounjaro recipe is built on **natural, whole ingredients** with scientifically backed health benefits. It is free from artificial additives, preservatives, or stimulants, making it a **safe and sustainable option** for those looking to improve their health.

With its **vibrant color, refreshing taste, and multi-faceted benefits**, the drink has gained traction among those looking for a natural approach to weight management, inflammation reduction, and overall wellness.

In the next chapter, we will explore how this drink plays a role in **weight loss, detoxification, and supporting metabolic health**, along with practical ways to incorporate it into your daily routine.

Chapter Two

How the Brazilian Mounjaro Drink Supports Weight Loss and Detoxification

The Science of Weight Loss and Detoxification

Weight loss is not just about cutting calories—it's about how the body processes and utilizes energy. Many people struggle with weight gain due to **slow metabolism, high inflammation levels, and poor digestion**. The Brazilian Mounjaro drink supports weight loss in a holistic way by targeting these issues at their core.

How the Key Ingredients Aid Weight Loss

1. Apple Cider Vinegar – A Natural Fat Burner

- Helps control **appetite and cravings**, leading to reduced calorie intake.

- Improves **insulin sensitivity**, allowing the body to use glucose more efficiently instead of storing it as fat.

- Boosts **fat oxidation**, meaning the body burns fat more efficiently for energy.

2. Lemon Juice – Detoxifying and Metabolism-Boosting

- Supports the **liver's natural detoxification** processes, which are essential for weight loss.

- The high vitamin C content boosts the immune system and **reduces inflammation** that can contribute to stubborn fat storage.

- Enhances hydration, helping to curb hunger and support digestion.

3. Butterfly Pea Flowers – Fighting Inflammation and Cravings

- High in **antioxidants**, which reduce inflammation and improve metabolism.

- Helps balance **blood sugar levels**, reducing spikes that can lead to increased fat storage and cravings.

- Supports **brain function and mental clarity**, which is crucial for staying motivated on a weight loss journey.

4. Honey – A Smart Energy Source

- Unlike refined sugars, honey provides a slow, steady energy release that **prevents blood sugar crashes**.

- Contains enzymes that improve **digestion and gut health**, leading to better nutrient absorption and metabolism regulation.

- Helps **reduce stress hormones** that can contribute to emotional eating and weight gain.

How the Brazilian Mounjaro Drink Supports Detoxification

- **Flushes out toxins:** Lemon juice and ACV help the liver process and remove harmful substances from the body.

- **Supports kidney function:** Helps to eliminate excess waste and prevent bloating.

- **Boosts digestion:** A healthy gut microbiome leads to improved metabolism and reduced inflammation.

- **Hydration and cleansing:** Drinking this beverage daily promotes hydration, which is essential for flushing toxins and maintaining a healthy weight.

Incorporating the Drink into Your Routine

- **Morning Boost:** Start your day with the drink to jumpstart your metabolism and curb cravings.

- **Before Meals:** Drinking it before meals helps control appetite and improve digestion.

- **Post-Workout:** The nutrients and hydration aid in muscle recovery and detoxification.

- **Daily Cleanse:** Consuming it consistently can lead to long-term benefits, including sustained weight loss and improved energy levels.

In the next chapter, we'll explore **how inflammation and gut health play a crucial role in sustainable wellness** and how the Brazilian Mounjaro drink contributes to a balanced, healthy body.

Chapter Three

Inflammation and Gut Health – The Key to Sustainable Wellness

Understanding the Link Between Inflammation and Weight Gain

Inflammation is a natural response by the body's immune system to injury, infection, or toxins. However, when inflammation becomes chronic, it can have serious negative effects on overall health, including weight gain. **Chronic inflammation can lead to insulin resistance, metabolic disorders, and increased fat storage, particularly around the abdominal area.** This is because inflammation disrupts the normal function of insulin, the hormone responsible for regulating blood sugar levels. When insulin function is impaired, the body stores more fat instead of using it for energy.

Additionally, systemic inflammation can cause hormonal imbalances that increase hunger signals and cravings for high-calorie, processed foods. This creates a cycle where poor dietary choices fuel inflammation, leading to further weight gain and difficulty losing excess fat. Reducing inflammation through diet and lifestyle changes can **restore metabolic balance, enhance fat burning, and improve overall health.**

The Role of Gut Health in Weight Loss

The gut microbiome—composed of trillions of bacteria and microorganisms—plays a critical role in metabolism, digestion, and immune function. A healthy gut supports nutrient absorption, reduces inflammation, and enhances metabolism, while an unhealthy gut can lead to bloating, sluggish digestion, and weight retention.

When harmful bacteria outnumber beneficial bacteria in the gut, it can result in **gut dysbiosis**, a condition linked to inflammation, weight gain, and digestive issues. Poor gut health can also **negatively impact the production of short-chain fatty acids (SCFAs), which help regulate appetite and energy balance.**

By improving gut health, the body can better process and eliminate waste, reduce cravings, and maintain stable energy levels. **A balanced gut microbiome has been associated with lower inflammation levels, improved fat metabolism, and enhanced insulin sensitivity, all of which are crucial for sustainable weight loss.**

How the Brazilian Mounjaro Drink Reduces Inflammation

The Brazilian Mounjaro drink is packed with ingredients that help reduce inflammation naturally. Each component contributes to fighting oxidative stress, restoring gut balance, and promoting metabolic health:

- **Butterfly Pea Flowers:** Rich in **anthocyanins and antioxidants**, these flowers help neutralize harmful free radicals that contribute to inflammation. They also support blood vessel function, improving circulation and nutrient delivery to the gut.

- **Apple Cider Vinegar (ACV):** Contains **acetic acid**, which has been shown to **reduce inflammatory markers** and promote a balanced gut microbiome by encouraging the growth of beneficial bacteria.

- **Lemon Juice:** A great source of **vitamin C**, which is a powerful antioxidant that fights inflammation and supports liver function to aid in detoxification.

- **Honey:** Has **antimicrobial and anti-inflammatory properties**, which soothe the gut lining and promote the growth of good bacteria.

- **Ginger:** Contains gingerol and shogaol, which help block enzymes like cyclooxygenase (COX-2) and lipoxygenase that produce inflammatory molecules in the body.

By drinking the Brazilian Mounjaro beverage daily, **you can actively support your body's ability to combat chronic inflammation, improve digestion, and regulate metabolism.**

The Role of Honey and Vinegar in Balancing Gut Bacteria

Apple cider vinegar and honey work synergistically to promote gut health by fostering a favorable environment for beneficial bacteria while inhibiting the growth of harmful microbes.

- **Apple Cider Vinegar:**

  - Lowers the pH in the gut, making it difficult for harmful bacteria to thrive.

  - Enhances digestion by stimulating the production of stomach acid and enzymes.

  - Reduces bloating and promotes smoother digestion by breaking down food more effectively.

- **Honey:**

  - Acts as a **prebiotic**, feeding the good bacteria in the gut and helping them flourish.

  - Contains **antioxidants and polyphenols** that reduce inflammation in the digestive tract.

  - Has antibacterial properties that help combat gut infections and imbalances.

Together, these ingredients **restore gut health, improve digestion, and support immune function,** making them a vital part of an anti-inflammatory lifestyle.

Anti-Inflammatory Meal Pairings with the Brazilian Mounjaro Drink

To maximize the benefits of the Brazilian Mounjaro drink, it is best to pair it with nutrient-dense, anti-inflammatory foods that work in harmony with its properties. Here are some meal pairings that complement its effects:

Breakfast: Gut-Healing Smoothie & Mounjaro Drink

- **Smoothie Ingredients:**

  - Greek yogurt (probiotic boost)

  - Blueberries (antioxidants and fiber)

  - Chia seeds (omega-3s and fiber)

  - Spinach (anti-inflammatory nutrients)

  - Almond milk (dairy-free alternative)

- **How It Helps:**

  - This smoothie is packed with probiotics, fiber, and antioxidants to promote digestion and gut health.

- ○ When paired with the Brazilian Mounjaro drink, it enhances detoxification and metabolic support.

Lunch: Grilled Salmon with Quinoa and Avocado

- **Meal Ingredients:**

  - ○ Grilled wild-caught salmon (rich in omega-3 fatty acids)

  - ○ Quinoa (fiber and plant-based protein)

  - ○ Avocado (healthy fats and potassium)

  - ○ Steamed broccoli (anti-inflammatory nutrients)

- **How It Helps:**

  - ○ Omega-3s in salmon help **reduce inflammation and support brain health.**

  - ○ Fiber-rich quinoa and avocado promote gut health and stable blood sugar levels.

  - ○ Pairing this meal with the Mounjaro drink enhances digestion and nutrient absorption.

Dinner: Stir-Fried Vegetables with Turmeric and Brown Rice

- **Meal Ingredients:**

  - ○ Mixed bell peppers, zucchini, and carrots (fiber and antioxidants)

- Garlic and turmeric (anti-inflammatory spices)

- Olive oil (healthy monounsaturated fats)

- Brown rice (fiber and complex carbohydrates)

- **How It Helps:**

  - The combination of fiber, antioxidants, and healthy fats reduces inflammation and supports gut health.

  - Turmeric and garlic work together to fight oxidative stress and enhance digestion.

  - The Mounjaro drink further aids digestion and supports liver detoxification.

Snacks: Nuts, Dark Chocolate, or Probiotic-Rich Yogurt

- **Snack Options:**

  - Handful of almonds and walnuts (healthy fats and protein)

  - Dark chocolate (70%+ cocoa, rich in polyphenols)

  - Coconut yogurt (probiotic benefits)

- **How It Helps:**

  ○ Nuts and dark chocolate provide anti-inflammatory compounds that support heart and brain health.

  ○ Probiotic yogurt enhances gut flora, which complements the digestive benefits of the Mounjaro drink.

The relationship between **inflammation, gut health, and weight management** is undeniable. By reducing chronic inflammation and promoting a balanced gut microbiome, **you can unlock sustainable weight loss and improved overall health.** The Brazilian Mounjaro drink is a powerful tool that supports digestion, regulates blood sugar, and enhances detoxification when combined with an anti-inflammatory diet.

In the next chapter, we'll dive deeper into **real-life success stories** of individuals who have transformed their health with the Brazilian Mounjaro drink and the specific strategies they used to sustain their results.

Chapter Four

Real-Life Success Stories – How the Brazilian Mounjaro Drink Transformed Lives

One of the best ways to understand the true power of the **Brazilian Mounjaro drink** is to hear from those who have incorporated it into their daily routines and seen remarkable transformations. From everyday individuals seeking a healthier lifestyle to Hollywood celebrities maintaining their peak physical condition, this drink has gained a loyal following.

Everyday People Who Achieved Life-Changing Results

Maria's Weight Loss and Energy Boost

Maria, a 45-year-old teacher from São Paulo, had been struggling with weight gain and constant fatigue. She tried numerous diets and workout plans, but nothing seemed to give her lasting results. After being introduced to the Brazilian Mounjaro drink by a friend, Maria decided to add it to her morning routine.

- Within **two weeks**, she noticed improved digestion and reduced bloating.

- By **two months**, she had lost **12 pounds** and felt significantly more energized throughout her busy teaching schedule.

- Maria also reported fewer cravings for processed foods and sweets, allowing her to maintain a healthier diet.

"I never imagined that a simple drink could make such a difference in my life. I feel lighter, healthier, and full of energy every day!"
– Maria C.

Jason's Transformation After Years of Digestive Issues

Jason, a 38-year-old IT professional from Los Angeles, had been struggling with **acid reflux, bloating, and inconsistent digestion** for years. His doctors recommended avoiding trigger foods, but nothing seemed to provide long-term relief. After learning about the gut-balancing properties of apple cider vinegar and honey in the Brazilian Mounjaro drink, he decided to give it a try.

- After **one month**, Jason reported fewer episodes of acid reflux and improved digestion.

- By **three months**, his bloating had significantly reduced, and he felt more comfortable after meals.

- He also experienced an unexpected **boost in mental clarity and focus** at work.

"This drink worked wonders for my gut health. I no longer suffer from uncomfortable bloating, and my energy levels have skyrocketed!"
-Jason L.

Hollywood Celebrities who Swear by the Ingredients in Brazilian Mounjaro Drink

The Brazilian Mounjaro drink has also caught the attention of Hollywood's biggest stars, who rely on natural health remedies to maintain their **physique, skin health, and overall well-being**. Several A-list celebrities have incorporated this beverage into their health routines for its anti-inflammatory and metabolism-boosting benefits.

Kelly Clarkson Weight Loss Journey

Renowned for her powerful vocals and candid personality, has recently shared insights into her weight loss journey. In a conversation with Whoopi Goldberg on *The Kelly Clarkson Show*, Kelly revealed that she utilized a medication to aid in her weight loss, clarifying that it was not Ozempic but another treatment that assists in breaking down sugar in the body.

Kelly emphasized that her decision to use medication was driven by health concerns, including being prediabetic, and a desire to improve her overall well-being. She also highlighted the importance of consulting with healthcare professionals to determine the best approach for individual health needs.

While Kelly did not specifically mention the Brazilian Mounjaro drink in her weight loss regimen, her openness about seeking effective methods to manage weight and health underscores the importance of personalized and informed approaches to wellness.

"Everybody thinks it's Ozempic. It's not," Kelly stated, *addressing common misconceptions about her weight loss methods.*

Her journey serves as a reminder that weight loss and health management are deeply personal and should be approached with care and professional guidance.

Jennifer Aniston's Secret to Ageless Glow

Known for her **glowing skin and toned figure**, Jennifer Aniston is a huge advocate for **natural, anti-inflammatory foods and drinks**. According to sources, she includes ingredients found in the Brazilian Mounjaro drink—such as **lemon, honey, and apple cider vinegar**—in her morning hydration routine.

- Helps detoxify the body and keep her metabolism active.

- Supports **radiant skin** by reducing inflammation and oxidative stress.

- Keeps digestion on track, which contributes to a **flat stomach** and lean physique.

*"I always start my day with a refreshing drink packed with antioxidants—it's the best way to wake up my body and skin." – **Jennifer A.***

Chris Hemsworth's Metabolism Hack

As an action star, **Chris Hemsworth** follows a strict diet and workout regimen to stay in peak physical shape. Apple cider vinegar and antioxidant-rich drinks like the Brazilian Mounjaro beverage have been part of his routine for **fat metabolism and digestion support**.

- Helps burn fat efficiently while maintaining **lean muscle mass**.

- Keeps his immune system strong during long filming schedules.

- Supports gut health, reducing bloating and improving energy levels.

*"Good nutrition is everything when it comes to fitness. I use natural remedies like lemon and apple cider vinegar to keep my metabolism in check." – **Chris H.***

Gwyneth Paltrow's Go-To Detox Drink

Well-known for her dedication to **clean eating and natural wellness**, **Gwyneth Paltrow** is a fan of drinks with detoxifying properties. Her health brand often highlights beverages that include **apple cider vinegar, lemon, and antioxidants**—all key components of the Brazilian Mounjaro drink.

- Helps keep digestion smooth and reduces bloating.

- Aids in detoxifying the liver and promoting skin health.

- Provides a **natural energy boost** without caffeine.

"I love drinks that help the body detox and recharge—it's all about balance and using nature's best ingredients." – ***Gwyneth P.***

In the next chapter, we will explore how **incorporating this drink into your daily routine can lead to long-term health benefits, and how to customize it for different needs and preferences.**

Chapter Five

Making the Brazilian Mounjaro Drink Part of Your Daily Routine

Why Consistency Matters

Incorporating the Brazilian Mounjaro drink into your daily routine can have profound effects on metabolism, digestion, inflammation, and overall wellness. However, **consistency is key**. While drinking it once or twice may provide short-term benefits, long-term health improvements require regular consumption. When paired with a balanced diet and healthy lifestyle, this drink can become a valuable part of a holistic wellness plan.

Best Times to Drink the Brazilian Mounjaro Beverage

1. Morning Boost: Kickstarting Your Metabolism

- Drinking the Mounjaro beverage in the morning can help jumpstart your metabolism for the day ahead.

- Apple cider vinegar aids in stabilizing blood sugar levels and reducing cravings.

- Lemon juice and butterfly pea flowers provide an antioxidant boost that energizes and detoxifies the body.

- Best paired with a high-protein breakfast such as scrambled eggs and avocado toast to sustain energy levels.

2. Pre-Meal Digestive Aid

- Consuming the drink 15-30 minutes before meals supports digestion by stimulating digestive enzymes and reducing bloating.

- Apple cider vinegar helps break down food more efficiently and promotes better nutrient absorption.

- Helps prevent post-meal sugar spikes, making it particularly beneficial for individuals managing blood sugar levels.

3. Post-Workout Recovery

- Hydration is critical after exercise, and the Mounjaro drink replenishes lost electrolytes.

- The anti-inflammatory properties of its ingredients help reduce muscle soreness and promote faster recovery.

- Pairs well with a post-workout snack like a protein smoothie or a bowl of Greek yogurt with honey and nuts.

4. Evening Cleanse and Relaxation

- Drinking this beverage in the evening can aid in digestion and prepare the body for restful sleep.

- The natural calming properties of butterfly pea flowers and honey can help soothe the nervous system.

- Apple cider vinegar supports detoxification processes that occur overnight, promoting better gut health by morning.

- Best paired with a light dinner consisting of leafy greens and lean proteins.

Variations of the Brazilian Mounjaro Drink

While the original recipe is already powerful, slight modifications can be made to **enhance benefits** or **suit different preferences**:

1. Immunity-Boosting Version

- **Add:** A dash of cayenne pepper.

- **Benefits:** Cayenne enhances circulation and metabolism.

2. Gut-Healing Blend

- **Add:** A teaspoon of aloe vera juice and a sprinkle of cinnamon.

- **Benefits:** Aloe vera soothes the digestive tract, while cinnamon helps balance blood sugar levels.

3. Energy-Enhancing Recipe

- **Add:** A teaspoon of matcha powder or green tea extract.

- **Benefits:** Provides a natural caffeine boost without causing jitters.

4. Cooling and Refreshing Version

- **Add:** Mint leaves and cucumber slices.

- **Benefits:** Perfect for hot days, mint aids digestion while cucumber hydrates the body.

Pairing the Drink with a Healthy Lifestyle

While the Brazilian Mounjaro drink is beneficial on its own, pairing it with a **nutrient-dense diet, regular physical activity, and stress management techniques** will yield the best results.

Here's how:

1. Nutrition

- Focus on whole, unprocessed foods rich in fiber, healthy fats, and lean proteins.

- Avoid excessive sugar, processed foods, and refined carbs that contribute to inflammation.

- Incorporate plenty of colorful vegetables and fruits to boost antioxidant levels.

2. Exercise

- Engage in regular movement, such as walking, yoga, or strength training.

- Exercise supports metabolic function and helps combat inflammation.

- Post-workout consumption of the Mounjaro drink aids in faster muscle recovery.

3. Stress Management

- Chronic stress contributes to inflammation and hormonal imbalances.

- Implement relaxation techniques such as meditation, deep breathing, or journaling.

- The calming effects of butterfly pea flowers in the Mounjaro drink can help alleviate stress-related inflammation.

Creating a Habit for Long-Term Success

Consistency is best achieved when habits become second nature. Here are some tips to make incorporating this drink into your routine **effortless**:

- **Prepare in Advance:** Make a batch and store it in the fridge for easy access.

- **Set Reminders:** Use phone alerts to remind you to drink it at optimal times.

- **Pair It with an Existing Habit:** For example, drink it while preparing breakfast or before your evening wind-down routine.

- **Keep It Fun:** Experiment with different variations to keep it interesting and aligned with your personal preferences.

The Brazilian Mounjaro drink is a simple yet powerful addition to a **healthy lifestyle**, offering metabolic, digestive, and anti-inflammatory benefits. By making it a part of your daily routine and complementing it with nutritious meals, movement, and mindfulness, you can **maximize its effects and support long-term health goals.**

The Takeaway: A Simple Drink with Powerful Results

Whether it's everyday people looking to **lose weight, improve digestion, or boost their energy** or celebrities aiming to maintain **youthful vitality and peak physical shape**, the Brazilian Mounjaro drink has proven to be an effective, all-natural addition to a wellness routine.

With its ability to **reduce inflammation, enhance metabolism, and support gut health**, this simple yet powerful drink has helped countless individuals **transform their health from the inside out**. We have explored the many benefits of the **Brazilian Mounjaro drink** and how it can support **weight loss, inflammation reduction, and overall wellness**. From its **science-backed ingredients** to real-life success stories, it's clear that this drink is more than just a passing health trend—it's a sustainable approach to long-term well-being.

How to Take the Next Step

If you're looking to improve your health naturally, start by integrating the **Brazilian Mounjaro drink** into your daily routine. Whether it's first thing in the morning, before meals, or post-workout, **consistency is the key** to seeing lasting results.

By making small changes—like swapping processed drinks for this **nutrient-packed elixir**—you're giving your body the tools it needs to function optimally.

Your Health, Your Journey

The path to wellness is not about quick fixes—it's about sustainable habits that nourish and strengthen your body from the inside out. With the **Brazilian Mounjaro drink**, you now have a simple, effective tool to help you along the way.

In the next and final chapter we reveal the recipe; cheers to a healthier, more vibrant you!

Chapter Six

The Brazilian Mounjaro Drink Recipe

Ingredients:

- **Water:** 500 ml (about 2 cups)

- **Dried Butterfly Pea Flowers:** 2 tablespoons

- **Honey:** 1 teaspoon

- **Fresh Ginger (optional):** 1 teaspoon, sliced

- **Lemon Juice:** 1 teaspoon

- **Apple Cider Vinegar:** 1 teaspoon

Instructions:

1. **Boil Water:** In a saucepan, bring 500 ml of water to a rolling boil.

2. **Add Ginger (Optional):** If using fresh ginger, add the slices to the boiling water to infuse flavor.

3. **Steep Butterfly Pea Flowers:** Remove the saucepan from heat and add 2 tablespoons of dried butterfly pea flowers. Let them steep for about 10 minutes to extract their vibrant color and flavor.

4. **Strain the Mixture:** After steeping, strain the liquid into a pitcher or large glass to remove the flowers (and ginger slices, if used).

5. **Add Honey, Lemon Juice, and Apple Cider Vinegar:** Stir in 1 teaspoon of honey, 1 teaspoon of lemon juice, and 1 teaspoon of apple cider vinegar. Mix well until the honey is fully dissolved.

6. **Observe the Color Change:** The addition of lemon juice will cause the deep blue tea to transform into a beautiful purple hue, enhancing its visual appeal.

7. **Serve:** You can enjoy this drink warm or chilled. For a cold beverage, allow it to cool to room temperature, then pour over ice cubes in a glass.

Optional Variations:

- **Citrus Twist:** Substitute lemon juice with lime juice for a different citrus flavor.

- **Herbal Infusion:** Add a sprig of fresh mint or basil during the steeping process for an added layer of flavor.

- **Spice It Up:** Include a pinch of cayenne pepper for a subtle kick and potential metabolism boost.

Bibliography

1.Harvard Health Publishing. "The Role of Gut Health in Weight Management and Inflammation." Retrieved from https://www.health.harvard.edu

2. National Institutes of Health (NIH). "Apple Cider Vinegar and Its Metabolic Benefits." Retrieved from https://www.nih.gov

3. Mayo Clinic. "Understanding the Connection Between Digestion, Inflammation, and Weight Loss." Retrieved from https://www.mayoclinic.org

4. Journal of Functional Foods. "Anthocyanins in Butterfly Pea Flower and Their Impact on Inflammation and Gut Microbiota."

5. WebMD. "The Science Behind Honey and Its Anti-Inflammatory Effects." Retrieved from https://www.webmd.com

6. People Magazine. "Jennifer Aniston's Daily Morning Routine for Health and Wellness." Retrieved from https://www.people.com

7. Men's Health. "Chris Hemsworth's Nutrition Secrets for Staying in Superhero Shape." Retrieved from https://www.menshealth.com

8. Goop. "Gwyneth Paltrow's Go-To Detox Drinks and Their Health Benefits." Retrieved from https://www.goop.com

9. Sky News *Kelly Clarkson addresses weight loss medication speculation*–Journal of Alternative and Complementary Medicine. "The Detoxifying and Antioxidant Properties of Lemon Juice." Retrieved from https://news.sky.com/story/kelly-clarkson-addresses-w eight-loss-medication-speculation-13135657?utm

10. ABC News *Kelly Clarkson recognizing on-screen image prompted weight loss journey. Retrieved from https://abcnews.go.com/GMA/Wellness/kelly-clarkson-recognizi ng-screen-prompted-weight-loss-journey/story?id=110214072&utm*

11. Women's Health Magazine *Kelly Clarkson addresses weight loss speculation. Retrieved from https://www.womenshealthmag.com/wei ght-loss/a46128448/kelly-clarkson-weight-loss/?utm*

12. Journal of Alternative and Complementary Medicine. "The Detoxifying and Antioxidant Properties of Lemon Juice."

13. National Center for Biotechnology Information (NCBI). "Effects of Apple Cider Vinegar on Blood Sugar Regulation and Metabolism."

Notes

Use this section as a journal. Keep track of additional recipes, and additional goals you have set for yourself.

_____

_____

_____

_____

_____

_____

_____

_____

_____

_____

_____

_____

_____

_____

_____

_____

_____

_____

_____

_____

_____

_____

_____

_____

_____

_____

_____

_____

_____

_____

_____

_____

_____

_____

_____

_____

_____

_____

_____

_____

_____

_____

_____

_____

_____

_____

_____

_____

_____

_____

_____

_____

_____

_____

_____

_____

_____

_____

_____

Thank you very much for your time. I wish you all the best! – H.M.

Made in United States
Orlando, FL
26 February 2025

58933558R00038